table of contents

yoga basics — 1
beer basics — 2
how to taste beer — 3

child's pose — 6
paired beer: wheat beer — 7

plank pose — 8
paired beer: kölsch — 9

down dog pose — 10
paired beer: gose — 11

chaturanga — 12
paired beer: pale ale — 13

side plank pose — 14
paired beer: robust porter — 15

pigeon pose — 16
paired beer: american ipa — 17

crow pose — 18
paired beer: american stout — 19

side crow pose   20
paired beer: imperial stout   21

triangle pose   22
paired beer: saison   23

warrior I pose   24
paired beer: brown   25

warrior II pose   26
paired beer: amber   27

warrior III pose   28
paired beer: rye ipa   29

hand to toe pose   30
paired beer: imperial ipa   31

chair pose   32
paired beer: blonde ale   33

revolved chair pose   34
paired beer: flanders   35

eagle pose   36
paired beer: belgian ipa   37

puppy pose   38
paired beer: pilsner   39

namaste   40

yoga basics

Yoga offers many physical benefits, such as increased flexibility, balance, strength, stamina and body alignment. Today's Western yoga practice has been adopted as a popular way of getting physically fit.

Through a series of breathing techniques and poses, also known as asanas, different types of yoga are formed. There are dozens of styles and practices of yoga — hatha, restorative, yin, vinyasa and hot, to name a few. Popular Western yoga classes are generally practiced with a series of asana flows where a combination of breath and motion lead to a peak pose.

There are four main categories of physical orientations that help define yoga postures: seated, standing, supine (lying face-up) and prone (lying face-down). Those four categories of postures can be grouped into pose types: balance, backbends, forward bends, core strength, hip openers, side bends, inversions, twists and arm balances.

In this book, you will find a variety of poses, from hip openers to arm balances. As your practice deepens, each of these asanas has many variations that can be adopted by the first timer or the seasoned yogi. Proper alignment is a key to the foundation of a yoga practice. Props such as blocks and straps are not just for beginners, as they can aid in balance and alignment.

Pairing beer and yoga is untraditional but both are about being a little adventurous and trying new things . This book is all about having an adventure!

beer basics

There are four main beer ingredients. These ingredients form the basis of all beer recipes and each one plays an integral part in the beer's character. There are numerous ingredients used, but these are the big four that make up almost every batch that is brewed today: water, yeast, malt and hops.

Water: makes up 90 to 95 percent of beer's content.

Yeast: converts sugar into CO_2 and alcohol, and also contributes to flavor.

Malt: grain is responsible for producing the fermentable sugars that yeast turns into alcohol. Malt adds more than alcohol to beer, as it influences flavor, aroma, body and color. There are many malted grains used in beer, but the most commonly used is barley.

Hops: balance the sweetness contributed from malt by adding bitterness. Hops added early in the brewing process will make it more bitter; hops added later in the brewing process will make it less bitter, and have more aroma and flavor.

Tip: International bitter units (IBU) is an approximate scale from 1-100. IBUs are not measured on the perceived bitterness of the beer, but the amount of isohumulone — the acid found in hops that gives beer its bitter bite. There are several methods to measure IBU.

There are many different types of beer. The two most common parent types are ales and lagers, both which contain many subtypes. Simply said, the main difference between ales and lagers is the yeast used in the brewing process.

Ales are "top-fermenting" and ferment at warmer temperatures for shorter periods of time. A few ale styles include stout, India pale ale, hefeweizen and amber.

Lagers are "bottom-fermenting" and ferment at cooler temperatures for longer periods of time. A few lager styles include Pilsner, bock, dunkel and helles.

how to taste beer

Tasting beer for most is an art and an acquired ability, much like wine. Quite often, people only drink "light" beer because they are intimidated by "heavy" beers which tend to be darker colors of ambers, porters and stouts — or are scared of trying a "hoppy" beer because of the bitter taste. Dark beers generally have caramel, chocolate, coffee, maple or spice flavors. Hoppy beers tend to be very crisp and have piney, floral, fruity or citrus notes (depending on the hop variety) — that sounds pretty tasty!

Tip: Alcohol by volume or ABV is used to measure how much alcohol is in an alcoholic beverage. Beers on average range from 3 to 13% ABV.

Pour: tilt the glass at a 45-degree angle and pour slowly. Choose a glass based on the beer's style (see more in "glassware" on the next page).

Look: pause and marvel at its greatness before you partake in it – what a beautiful beer! Raise the beer in front of you, describe its color, its head (foam on top of the beer) and its consistency (still, uncarbonated, slightly carbonated, sparkling). What do you see in its appearance? *Color, head, carbonation levels, clarity.*

Agitate: swirl your beer (as you would with wine). This will pull out aromas, stimulate carbonation and test head retention.

Smell: breathe through your nose with one deep inhale. What aromas do you smell? *Chocolate, citrus, floral, spices.*

Taste: after smelling the beer, breathe out through your nose during the tasting process. Sip the beer and resist swallowing immediately. What do you taste? *Sweet, salty, sour, bitterness.* Observe the mouthfeel. How does it feel on your tongue? *Carbonated, crisp/dry, rich.*

Temperature: the temperature a beer is served at has an impact on taste. Beer served at very cold temperatures will impact things like carbonation and aroma, and it will numb the taste buds.

> *Tip: Try tasting the beer after it warms a bit (just a little — not too much). Really cold beer tends to mask some of the flavors. As a beer warms, its true flavors will come through and become more pronounced.*

Generally speaking, higher alcohol or more complex beers should be served at higher temperatures, while lower alcohol or lower complexity beers are better served at lower temperatures. The color of beer can also be a rough indicator of serving temperature. A lighter beer will do better at lower temps, and darker beer will do better at warmer temps. Your preference will always trump the recommended temperature, but the optimal temperature of beer is between 40 and 60 degrees Fahrenheit.

Glassware: in this book, you will find that each beer has unique glassware for its style. Why is this? As soon as beer hits a glass, factors like aroma, color, head and taste are altered and have an influence on your beer drinking experience. Therefore, glassware has been made to complement different beer styles. While it is a good idea to use glassware designed for a particular style of beer, pouring a stout into a mug or a saison into a pint glass is not going to ruin your beer or experience. Keep it simple and enjoy!

Brew & Asana: A BeerSnobChick's Guide to Beer and Yoga is my attempt to spread my love of craft beer and yoga to you by introducing yoga poses and pairing each one with a delicious brew. Easier, less complex poses are paired with lighter bodied, less complex brews, while more advanced poses are paired with more robust, complex brews. Cheers!

Tip: Tasting many beers at once will have an effect on your sensory perception. Taste brews with less alcohol content, less flavor and lighter color first. Follow up with brews with higher alcohol content, more flavor and a darker color.

child's pose

bring bum to heels

lengthen tailbone

lengthen neck

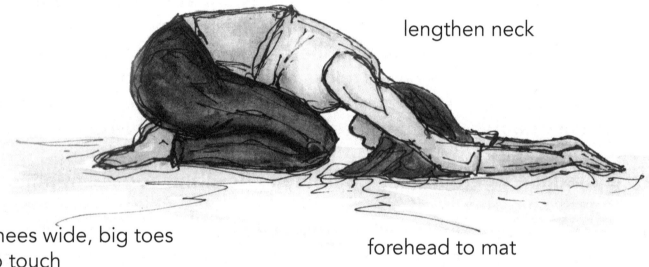

knees wide, big toes
to touch

forehead to mat

Tip: *Begin with your knees as wide as possible, toes to touch. Sit up straight and lengthen through the spine, then through the top of your head. As you exhale, bend forward, with your torso between your thighs. Broaden your upper back, soften your lower back. Extend your arms, palms facing down. If you have a shoulder injury, bring your arms back to rest alongside your thighs with your palms facing up. Child's pose will help remove tension in your back, shoulders, arms and neck.*

wheat beer

can be made with
ale or lager yeast

pale to golden in color

light to medium body

cloudy or hazy if
unfiltered

moderate in bitterness
10-35 IBU

often served with a
lemon wedge

alcohol by volume 3.5-6%

Beginner Pairing: *Child's pose is a relaxing pose, paired well with light, refreshing, easy drinking wheat beer.*

7

plank pose

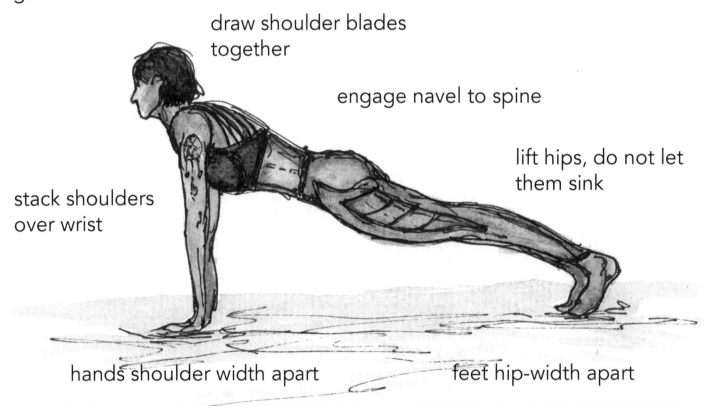

gaze forward

draw shoulder blades together

engage navel to spine

lift hips, do not let them sink

stack shoulders over wrist

hands shoulder width apart

feet hip-width apart

Tip: *Begin with hands shoulder width apart, press palms firmly into the mat. Engage the core and power through the thighs, draw shoulder blades together and down the back. Do not let the back start to "banana." If you are having trouble keeping the hips lifted, place knees on the ground for extra support.*

kölsch

slight, minimal head

very pale in color

light to medium body

malt character, dry and
crisp in flavor

medium to slightly
assertive bitterness
18-28 IBU

first brewed in
Köln, Germany

alcohol by volume 4.5-5.5%

Beginner Pairing: *Plank pose is foundational, while Kölsch is stable, slightly assertive and drinkable.*

down dog pose

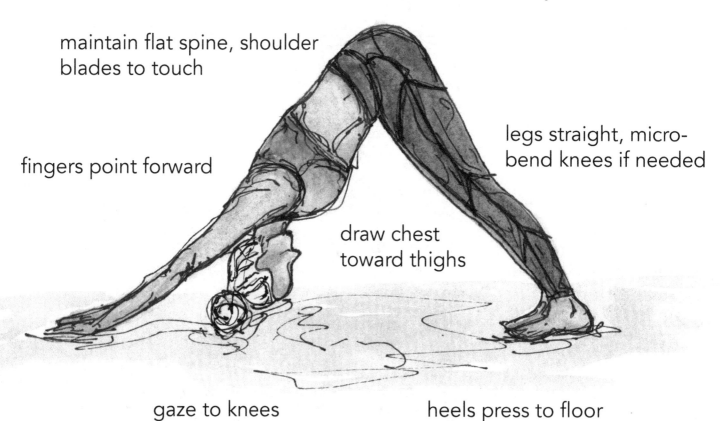

tailbone to the sky

maintain flat spine, shoulder blades to touch

legs straight, micro-bend knees if needed

fingers point forward

draw chest toward thighs

gaze to knees

heels press to floor

Tip: *To successfully set up down dog, the proper alignment comes from plank pose. Start in plank pose, lift the hips, do not shorten stance. Draw the heels to the mat. The goal is a flat spine in a "V" shape. If you cannot straighten legs, bend knees as much as you need to maintain a flat spine.*

gose

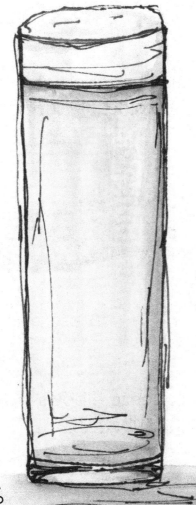

frothy head

cloudy yellow or straw to medium amber in color

light to medium body

unfiltered wheat, spice, herbal, floral or fruity aromas

low bitterness
10-15 IBU

old German style, refreshing, sharp and crisp

alcohol by volume 4-5.5%

Beginner Pairing: *Down dog is a foundational pose best paired with a flavorful and crisp, easy drinking gose.*

chaturanga pose

gaze to the tip
of nose

lengthen through
the spine

shift weight
forward, reach
through heels

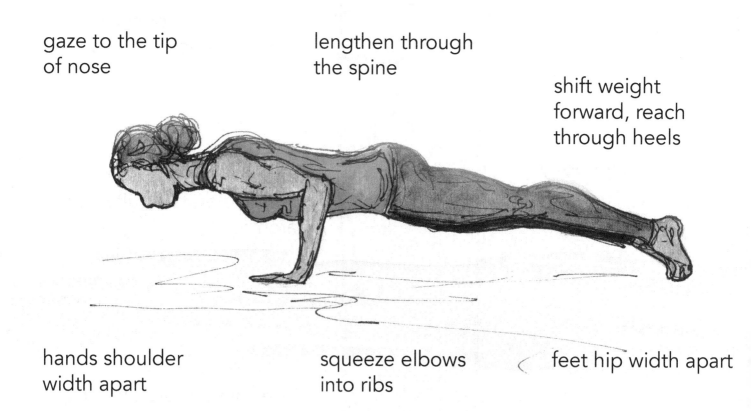

hands shoulder
width apart

squeeze elbows
into ribs

feet hip width apart

Tip: *Begin in plank pose. On an exhale, shift forward with the toes, bend the elbows, bring arms to a 90-degree angle. Keep the heart at elbow height. If you find that the shoulders are dipping down, drop to your knees for support. Hold for a couple breaths, push back up into plank pose or down dog pose.*

pale ale

medium head

golden to light amber in color

medium body

inspired by the classic English style ale

light to pungent bitterness
30-50 IBU

balance of malt and hops

alcohol by volume 4-7%

floral, fruity, citrus and piney aromas

Intermediate Pairing: *Chaturanga is a foundational strong pose best paired with a balanced malt and hoppy pale ale.*

side plank pose

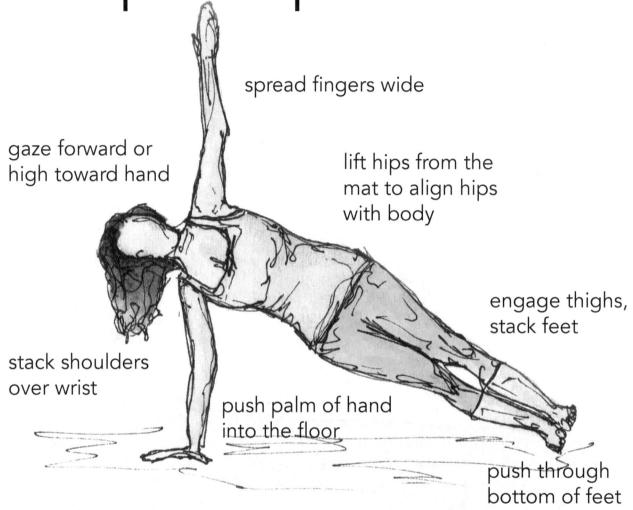

spread fingers wide

gaze forward or
high toward hand

lift hips from the
mat to align hips
with body

stack shoulders
over wrist

engage thighs,
stack feet

push palm of hand
into the floor

push through
bottom of feet

Tip: *Begin in plank pose. Plant your palm onto the mat and shift your weight. Stack your shoulders, hips and feet. Lift your hips to reach this pose to its fullest. Until you have enough strength to fully support your body weight, bring your bottom knee and shin to the mat.*

robust porter

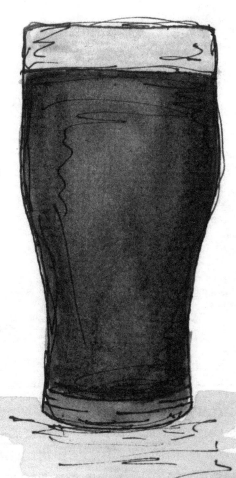

off-white to light tan head

light to medium body

range of bitterness
25-50 IBU

alcohol by volume
4.8-6.5%

light brown to dark
malty color

evident hop bitterness

cocoa with caramel and
roasted malty sweetness

some aged in bourbon
or whiskey barrels

Intermediate Pairing: *Side plank is a powerful arm strengthener that is perfectly balanced with a robust porter.*

pigeon pose

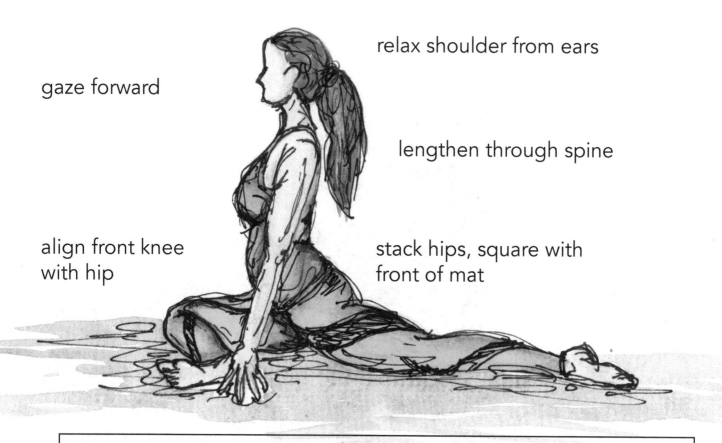

gaze forward

relax shoulder from ears

lengthen through spine

align front knee with hip

stack hips, square with front of mat

Tip: *From down dog pose, draw your knee to your torso. Place the outside of your foot, shin and knees on the mat. Keep fingertips slightly wider than your torso, press through your fingertips as you lift your torso away from your thigh to lengthen the front of your body. Your torso should be parallel or square to the front of the mat. Engage your core muscles to square your hips, drawing the top of the back hip toward the mat. Do not put your weight onto the outside of the forward hip (bent leg).*

american ipa

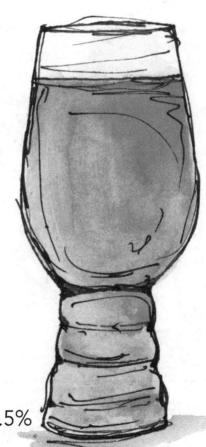

thin to medium head

range from very pale to
reddish-amber in color

moderate to medium
body

floral, fruity, tropical,
citrus and piney
character

moderate to high
bitterness
40-100 IBU

balanced malt
backbone

alcohol by volume 5.5-7.5%

IPA is short for India
Pale Ale

Intermediate Pairing: *Pigeon pose has many modifications from beginner to advanced, and is best paired with vast variations of an American IPA.*

crow pose

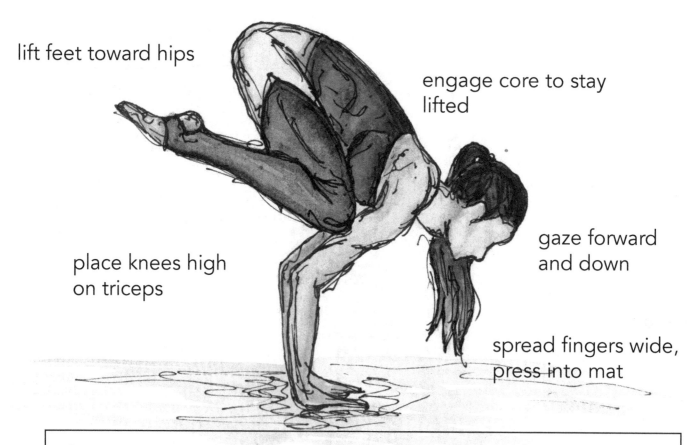

lift feet toward hips

engage core to stay lifted

place knees high on triceps

gaze forward and down

spread fingers wide, press into mat

Tip: *From a squat position, bring your palms to the mat. Lift onto the balls of your feet as you lean forward. Press your shins against the back of your upper arms. Draw knees in as close to your underarms as possible. Draw your abs in. Round your back, tuck tailbone in toward your heels. Lift your feet off the floor and draw your heels toward your bum. If it is difficult to lift both feet at the same time, lift one foot, then the other. Practice.*

american stout

long-lasting full head

medium to heavy body

wide range of bitterness
35-75 IBU

alcohol by volume 5-7%

dark brown to black
in color

notes of coffee or
chocolate added to
complement roasted
flavors

some aged in bourbon or
whiskey barrels

Advanced Pairing: Crow is an arm balance gateway pose, and perfectly paired with the complexity of an American stout and its flavor variations.

side crow pose

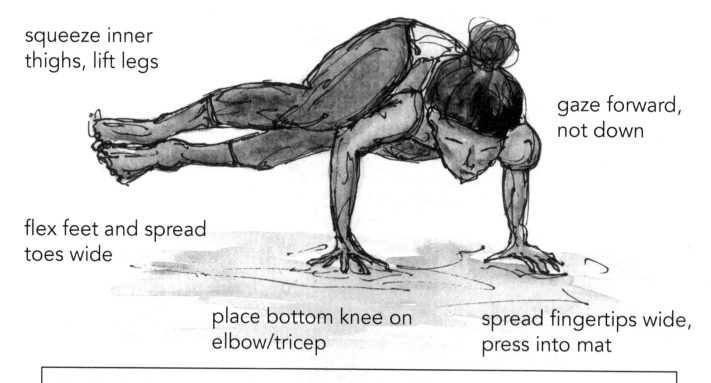

engage core to stay lifted

draw shoulder blades together

squeeze inner thighs, lift legs

gaze forward, not down

flex feet and spread toes wide

place bottom knee on elbow/tricep

spread fingertips wide, press into mat

Tip: Begin in a squatted position with knees together, take your left elbow to the outside of the right knee. Maximize rotation, come onto the balls of the feet, sink your hips deeply. Begin to float both feet off the floor, draw heels toward your bum. Stack knees directly on top of one another, lift shins parallel to the floor. Lead with the heart, press down evenly through your palms. Refine the pose by working to straighten the arms over time.

imperial stout

long-lasting head

full to heavy body

moderate to high
bitterness
50-90 IBU

alcohol by volume 7-12%

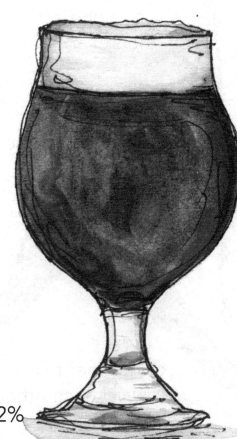

dark brown to
black in color

rich, roasted flavors

higher hop levels and
more residual sweetness

many are barrel aged,
mostly in bourbon and/or
whiskey barrels

Advanced Pairing: *Side crow is a twist on crow pose, and best paired with a rich, more flavorful and intense imperial stout.*

triangle pose

gaze toward fingertips, fingers to the sky

open chest, roll rib cage to the sky, rotate from the core

stack shoulders, draw shoulder blades down toward midline

lengthen through the spine

heels aligned, back foot parallel with mat

both legs straight

draw inner thighs toward each other

Tip: *This pose is prime for a prop block. If you cannot extend both legs straight, place a block next to the inside of the front ankle. Soften the knee by micro-bending it, which aids in protecting the hamstrings and lower back from overstretching.*

saison

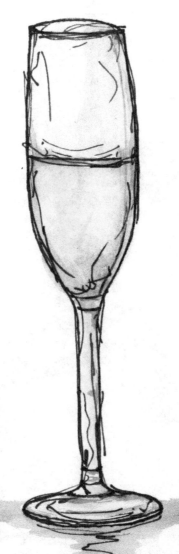

fruity aroma and flavor

light to medium body

low to medium in
bitterness 20-40 IBU

alcohol by volume 4.4-8%

pale straw to light gold in
color

mild to moderate tartness,
lots of spice

commonly called
"farmhouse ale"

traditionally brewed in
the winter and consumed
throughout the summer

Intermediate Pairing: Triangle pose is a stable, stress relieving pose best paired with a light and flavorful summer brew like a saison.

warrior I pose

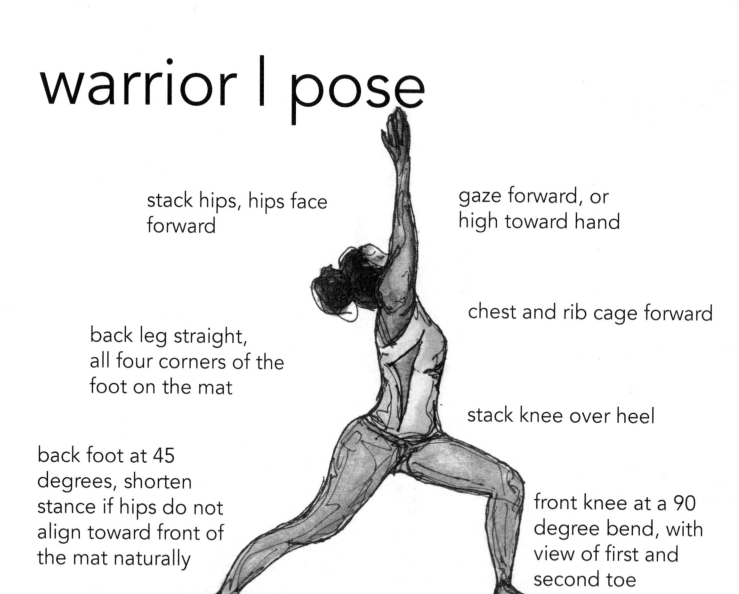

stack hips, hips face forward

gaze forward, or high toward hand

back leg straight, all four corners of the foot on the mat

chest and rib cage forward

stack knee over heel

back foot at 45 degrees, shorten stance if hips do not align toward front of the mat naturally

front knee at a 90 degree bend, with view of first and second toe

Tip: *From down dog pose turn your back toes to the left 45 degrees, toes pointing toward the top corner of the mat. Step front foot forward between the hands, a little to the right. Square the hips — they should be parallel to the top of the mat. Shorten your stance if you cannot get the outer edge of the foot and heel on the ground. Reach the arms up.*

brown ale

light head

dark amber to brown in color

light to medium body

notes of coffee or roasted nut

moderate in bitterness 20-45 IBU

roasted malt, caramel and chocolate characteristics

alcohol by volume 4-8%

Intermediate Pairing: *Warrior I is a stability pose with subtle details, much like the brown ale and its many variations.*

warrior ll pose

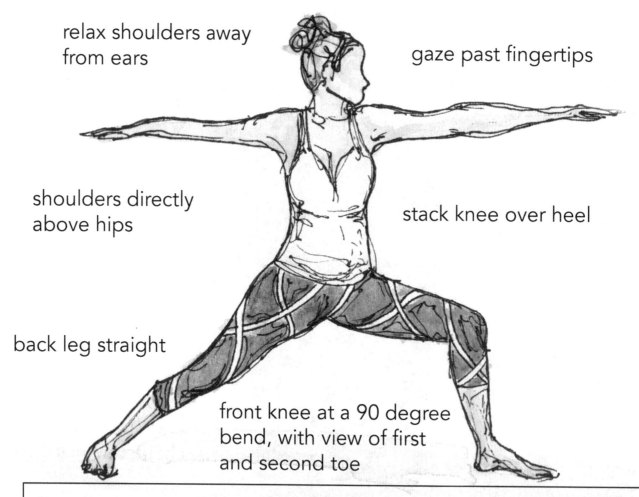

relax shoulders away
from ears

gaze past fingertips

shoulders directly
above hips

stack knee over heel

back leg straight

front knee at a 90 degree
bend, with view of first
and second toe

Tip: *Turn back foot 90 degrees so toes are parallel to the back of the mat.
The heel of your front foot should align to the middle of the arch of your
back foot. The front knee is bent at 90 degrees and stacked directly over
the ankle. Knee should not be in front of the ankle. Open through the hips.*

amber

light to medium head

amber to deep red in color

light to medium body

balanced with toasted malt characters

low to medium in bitterness
25-45 IBU

light fruitiness, moderate citrus hops

caramel and nutty character

alcohol by volume 4-7%

Intermediate Pairing: *Warrior II is a powerful and energizing pose and perfectly paired with a moderately hoppy and balanced amber brew.*

warrior III pose

leg straight, lift
parallel to mat

relax neck

arms straight

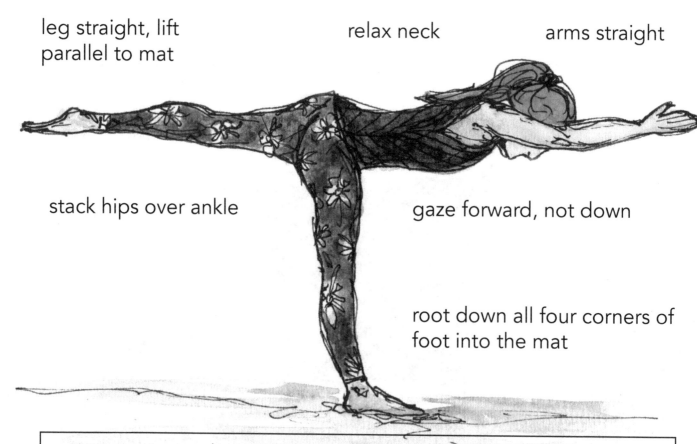

stack hips over ankle

gaze forward, not down

root down all four corners of
foot into the mat

Tip: With your front toes pointing to the front of the mat, slightly bend your
rooted leg. Find balance and strength in the front leg. With a flat back, draw
the back leg up. Turn the pinky toe of the lifted leg down toward the floor
so the hips are level, torso parallel to the floor. Engage your thigh muscles
and straighten your standing leg. Slowly extend your arms forward to the
front of the mat, align with the ears.

rye ipa

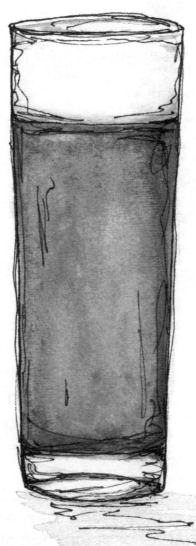

light head

light brownish-red in color

light to medium body

rye adds spicy and/or tangy, sour-like characteristics

moderate in bitterness 50-75 IBU

notable amount of rye grain

alcohol by volume 5.5-8%

often called a "RyePA"

Advanced Pairing: *Warrior III is a strong and balanced pose paired best with a dynamic and robust rye IPA.*

hand to toe pose

gaze opposite of
extended foot

broaden collar
bones

root all four corners of
foot into the mat

engage core

grab big toe with index and
middle fingers

first extend leg
forward, gain balance,
then open leg to
outside

Tip: *Begin in standing position with your feet together and arms at your sides. Shift your weight to the rooted foot, draw opposite knee up into the torso. On an exhalation, grab toes or outer edge of the foot, gently extend leg forward. Keep both hips squared forward and keep your spine straight. Straighten the knee as much as possible. If you are steady, open the hips and swing the extended leg out to the side.*

imperial ipa

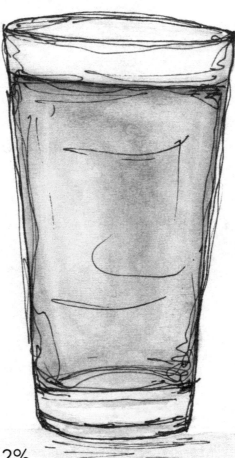

pale to golden in color

long-lasting head

high malty and
alcoholic characteristics

medium to full body

double or triple hopped

high in bitterness
65-100 IBU

often called "double
IPA" or "IIPA"

alcohol by volume 7.6-12%

Advanced Pairing: *Hand to toe is a challenging and invigorating pose that is best paired with the complex and intense imperial IPA.*

chair pose

spread fingers wide

extend arms, elbows to ears

flat back, elongate spine

navel to spine

tuck pelvis under body to remove the arch in back

bring weight into heels so that all 10 toes are visible, knees not to extend past toes

squat down

knees and toes to touch

Tip: *Stand with feet hip-distance apart. Raise arms above head, bend at the knees, thighs parallel to the mat. Draw the navel to the spine. Draw your shoulder blades down, reach your elbows toward your ears. Shift your weight into your heels so you can wiggle your toes. Spread your shoulder blades apart, palms face each other.*

blonde ale

medium white head

pale straw to deep golden in color

light body

known for simplicity, very balanced

moderate in bitterness 15-25 IBU

dry and sweet finish

often called "golden" ale

alcohol by volume 4-7%

Beginner Pairing: *Chair pose is a foundational powerful pose that is best paired with a more simplistic easy drinking blonde ale.*

revolved chair pose

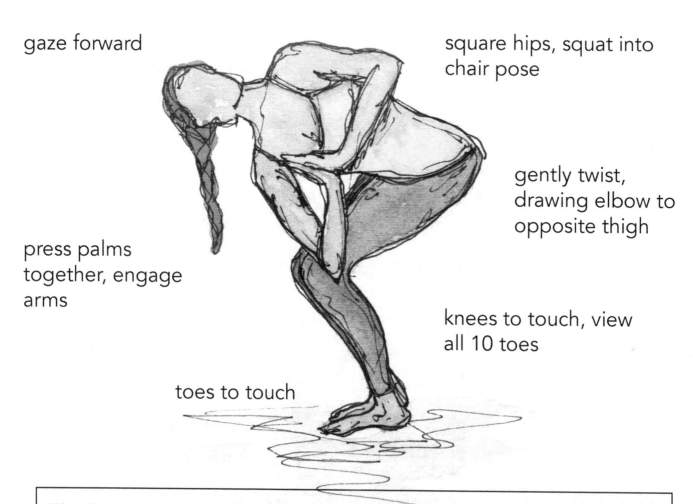

gaze forward

square hips, squat into chair pose

gently twist, drawing elbow to opposite thigh

press palms together, engage arms

knees to touch, view all 10 toes

toes to touch

Tip: *Start in chair pose, press palms together, engage your core. Gently twist and draw your elbow to the opposite thigh. To protect your knee joints, do not let one knee slide in front of the other. Keep knees parallel or even. Do not move knees over toes.*

flanders red

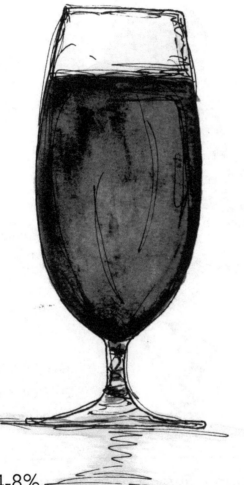

light head

reddish-brown in color

light body

cherry-like, plum, fig and raisin notes

low bitterness
5-18 IBU

oak or wood like characteristics

alcohol by volume 4.4-8%

very distinct and complex, sour or tart

Intermediate Pairing: *Revolved chair is a twist on chair pose and best paired with the delicious and complex Flanders red.*

eagle pose

press shoulders
away from ears

squeeze arms
together, lift elbows
toward the sky

long flat back,
engage core

elbows and knees
in line

squeeze legs together

press weight into
all four corners of
grounded foot

Tip: Begin in standing position. Sweep right arm under left at the elbows. Connect the palms if available. Shift weight to right foot. Squat into chair pose, lift opposite grounded leg, cross it as high as possible over your thigh. Square the hips. Do not lean forward and hunch over the knees and toes. For stability, squeeze legs and arms together.

belgian ipa

light gold to amber in color

billowy and large off-white head

slightly to quite cloudy

light to medium body

smooth and sweet maltiness, notes of caramel or toast

moderate to high in bitterness
50-90 IBU

spicy and clove-like, along with banana aroma and flavor

alcohol by volume 6-9.5%

Advanced Pairing: *Eagle pose is a strong endurance pose that meets its match with an unwavering and complex Belgian IPA.*

puppy pose

stack hips over knees,
knees hip distance apart

lengthen through the spine,
shoulders away from ears

spread fingers wide

align feet with
knees

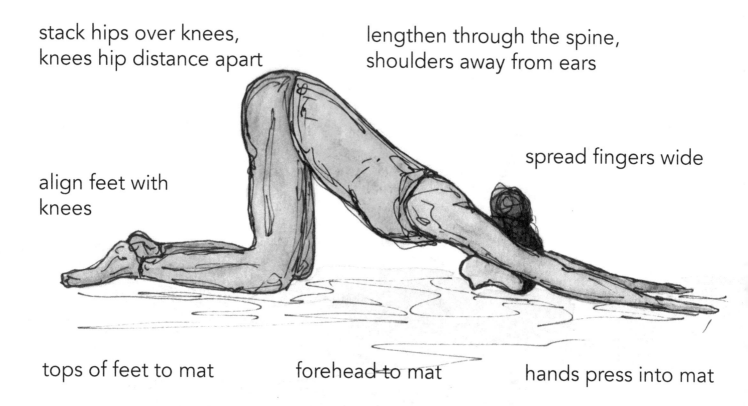

tops of feet to mat

forehead to mat

hands press into mat

Tip: *Start on all fours, shoulders stacked over wrists, hips stacked over knees, tops of the feet to the mat. Slowly walk your hands out in front of you, lowering your chest down toward the ground. Press the palms of your hands to the mat, and lift the elbows and forearms away from the ground. Lengthen your spine in both directions.*

pilsner

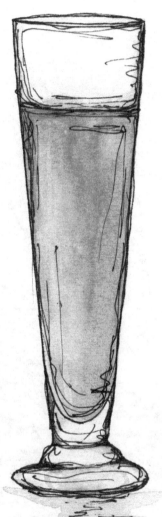

dense and rich head

light to medium body

moderate in bitterness
25-40 IBU

alcohol by volume 4-5.5%

light straw to golden in color

sharp hop bitterness

one of the most popular
styles of lagers

often spelled Pilsener or
spoken in slang as "Pils"

Beginner Pairing: *Puppy pose is a tension release pose that is fantastically paired with an easy drinking, crisp Pilsner.*

namaste

While combining yoga and beer is a bit of a stretch, it brings a unique harmony of a physical workout and social fellowship. Try something new, make it your own and have a new adventure! Namaste with a twist!

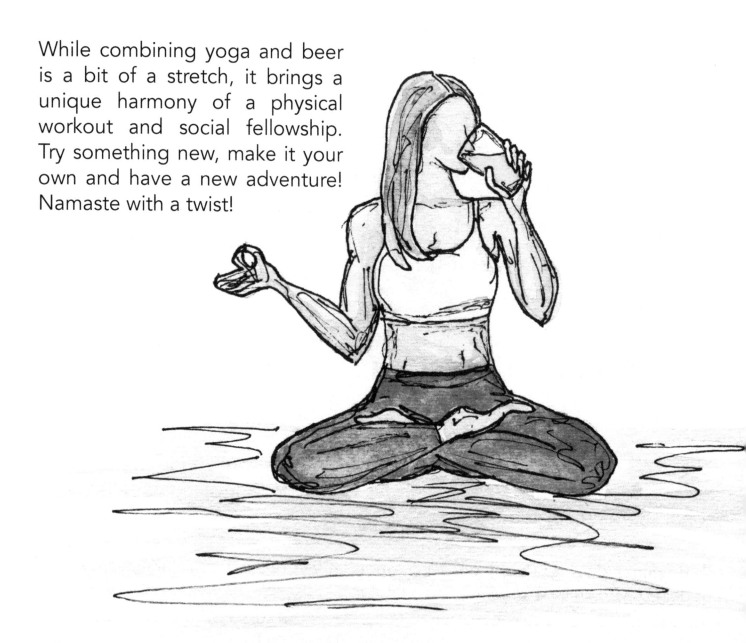

CPSIA information can be obtained
at www.ICGtesting.com
Printed in the USA
LVHW06s2339100918
589764LV00009B/24/P